Foreword

Having had the opportunity to look at the pictures in this book, I can understand where they are coming from. Why? Because I have got Vascular Dementia and it's not always easy to put into words that we cannot communicate with you. I do believe that this book will help to get the message across for people to understand about dementia and what we are going through.

They say a picture can say a thousand words and for us this is very true. So you need to look at the pictures and see what they are trying to tell you. I have looked through them and the one that stands out for me is "Human beings 1 Tin of beans 0" as it shows the dedication that people have to helping us. Take time to look and find the one that has special meaning for you.

Live your life as your life is for living –
Adventure before Dementia.

Dr Trevor Jarvis EDE BEM

A few words from the Author...

Dementia has long been the elephant in the room - often too big to ignore yet we still hoover around it...

In the pub, people would make jokes about Alzheimer's disease. I thought "they'd never do that if someone had cancer," then I realised that if they knew more they would think again.

I lost my Grandmother with dementia and, in caring ceaselessly for her, my own Mother was taken early. My Mother-in-Law was diagnosed at 59. Our lives are now all about

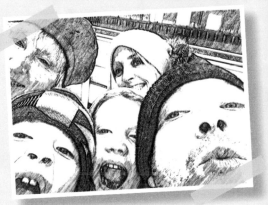

supporting her as a family.

Dementia is an uninvited guest. It does not discriminate and is often merciless, but amongst all of the tears and echoes of "Why me?" there is still laughter to be heard. A siege mentality often results in tighter relationships, celebration of small mercies and a strong family bond.

In the past few years I have worked with spies, FA Cup winners, ballroom dancers and bomber pilots all now with dementia. I go round many care homes working with care staff and have realised that to see only a person's dementia is like looking at their shadow and not talking to them. We should always remember which came first - the person, not dementia.

I wanted a book that captures the frustration and challenges faced by individuals, families and care staff. A book that children could read and understand. I wanted to show that dementia can affect us all and for people to empathise.

May this book deliver both the laughter and the tears. It is simple and free from jargon. I hope amid the sparing use of words and pictures it leaves room for your own feelings and emotions to help you better understand dementia and show others just how much you care.

You are not alone.

Never be afraid or too proud to ask for help.

We are better together.

thank you...

With this little book I have achieved an ambition I never realised I had.

Thank you to the love of my life Em for being a wonderful wife, mother and an invaluable daughter.

To Liz, Annie, Billy, Dad, Anna, Lulu the greyhound and Johnny for your ceaseless support.

I must thank Richard Hawkins and all at Hawker Publications for believing in my idea from the outset and finally to Chris Mitchell who turned this teacher into a student of every person I meet in the world of dementia care.

I realise people who care have one thing in short supply - time - so

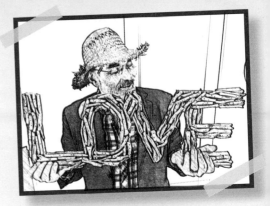

this is a short, simple book that cuts straight to the chase without meandering. Many books about dementia have the dubious quality that once you put them down you never pick them up again.

I'd like to think this little book will do the opposite and allow room for the conversations you've been afraid to have.

May your thoughts write the rest.

From the mouths of babes...

My little girl aged 10 stood on York Theatre Royal stage at 'A Night To Remember' - a concert for the Alzheimer's Society - and told 850 adults about 'Nana'. Proud doesn't even come close to how I felt.

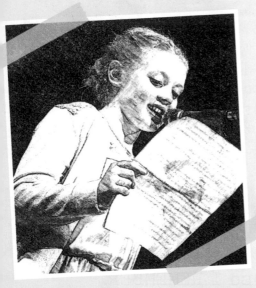

"Sometimes grown ups don't understand the important stuff."

"Before Nana I didn't know what Dementia was. I hadn't heard of Alzheimer's."

"Lots of people think Dementia only affects much older people in their 80s and 90s. My Nana was 58."

"The day Nana was diagnosed was the day we ALL got it."

"Families get dementia not just

the person with it.
Together is the only way
forward. Dementia is a
TEAM game."

"Nana still looks the same."

"We still sing in the
street, walk Lulu the crazy
greyhound, laugh together,
feed the birds, dance to
the radio and have girly
sleepovers where I am allowed
to stay up much later than Dad
lets me and watch programmes
I want to watch no matter how
dreadful."

"We can only help somebody if
we KNOW what the problem is."

"Once Nana was diagnosed as
having Alzheimer's, we knew
what we were dealing with."

"But life does not stop with
Alzheimer's."

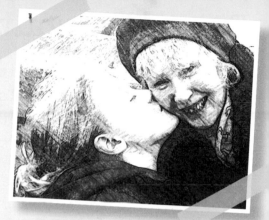

"Since diagnosis Nana has
danced on stage at 'Priscilla,
Queen of the Desert', met Bryan
Ferry and we visited New York
together as a family."

"Nana is still amazing.
Nana is still fun.
Nana can still ice-skate
backwards.
Nana is still my Nana.
But Nana forgets..."

SO I REMEMBER.

Dear Dementia,
We didn't invite you into our family
but you're here now.
We could focus totally on you
but we're going to focus on Nana instead.

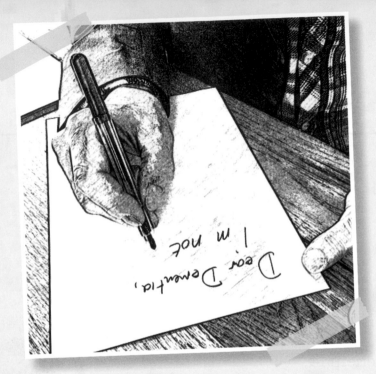

Dear Dementia,
I have you
You don't have me!

(With thanks to Chris Roberts)

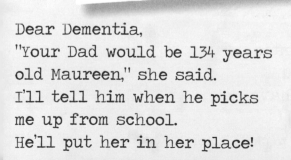

Dear Dementia,
"Your Dad would be 134 years
old Maureen," she said.
I'll tell him when he picks
me up from school.
He'll put her in her place!

Dear Dementia,
Mum carried me for 9 months,
Fed me, kept me safe.
She taught me right from wrong.
She'd have taken a bullet for me.
Every day of her life.
It's not YOU versus MUM.
It's YOU versus US!

Dear Dementia,
I wish **everybody**
would LISTEN
instead of telling
me what I want!

Dear Dementia,

I've just polished
off 6 walnut whips

Nothing to do
with you

I just love
walnut whips !

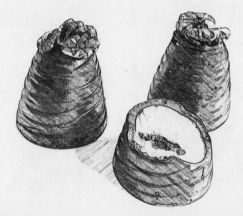

Dear Dementia,
My daughter's
exhausted.
Am I the reason
she's so tired?
Or is it you?
By all means
come for me
but please leave
her alone.

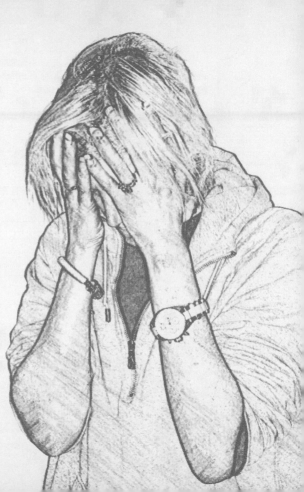

Dear Dementia,
My husband's gone.
Never had children.
It's just YOU AND ME
Together
Alone...

Personal announcements

to place an announcement phone **01904 676767**

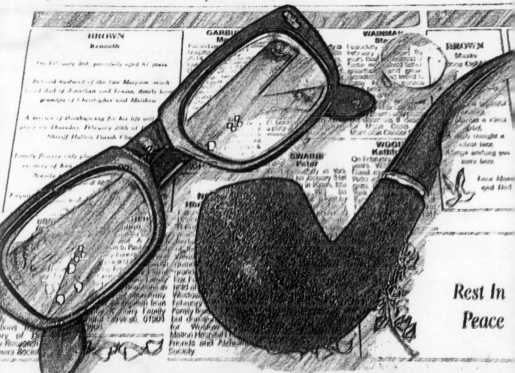

Rest In

Peace

Dear Dementia,
Everybody finishes my sentences.
Every night I'm left with a
bagful of unused full stops.

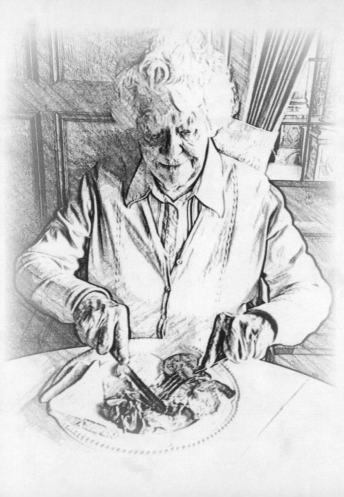

Dear Dementia,
I was a strict
vegetarian all
my life until
you came along
and now I've
discovered
bacon!

Dear Dementia,
Nana forgets,
so I remember.

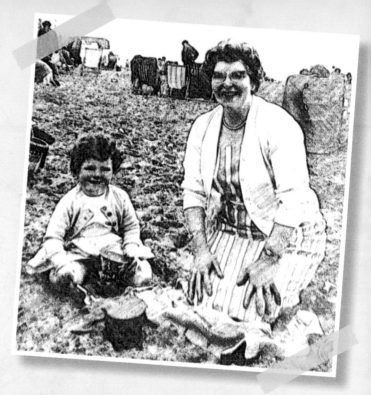

Dear Dementia,
Some days I feel like throwing in the towel and giving up. But then I think what if the shoe was on the other foot, how would Mum care for me?

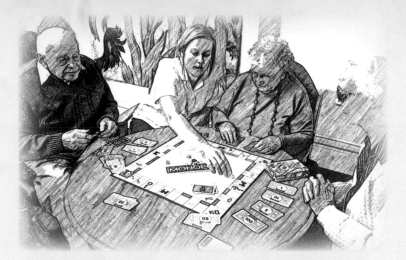

Dear Dementia,
This lass could get more money
stacking shelves in the supermarket
but we're so pleased she cares
for us instead

Human beings   1
Tins of beans 0

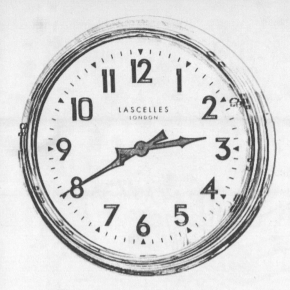

Dear Dementia,

You've turned my clock into a round picture on the wall.

I still have "o'clock" and "half past".

Please leave me with those...

Time is precious

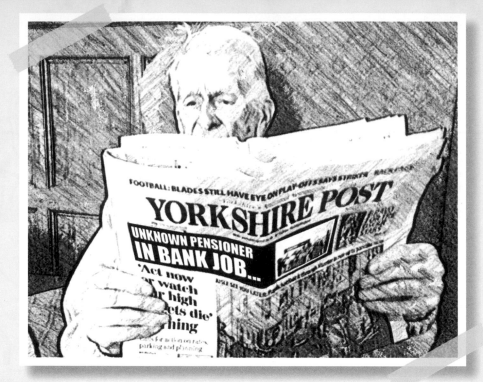

Dear Dementia,
I've looked at activities in care homes and
activities in prisons... I'm off to rob a bank!

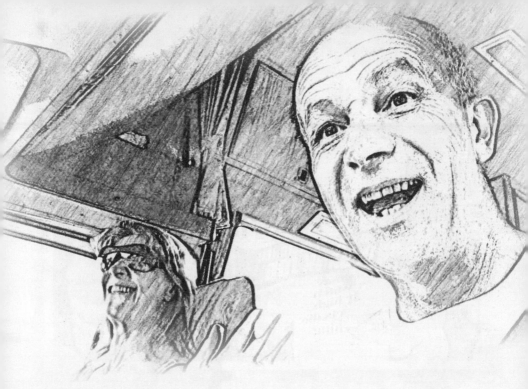

Dear Dementia,
I'm so glad my wife celebrates what's left of me and doesn't dwell on what you've taken.

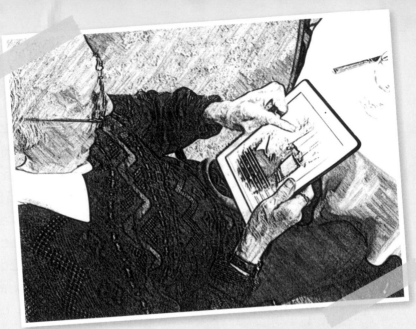

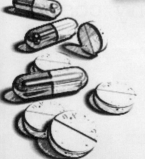

Dear Dementia,
So I can take this tablet anywhere,
it stores all my photos and songs,
I can talk to my son in
Australia on it and there are
no side effects?

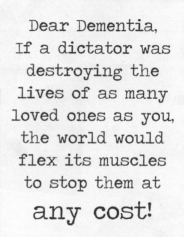

Dear Dementia,
If a dictator was destroying the lives of as many loved ones as you, the world would flex its muscles to stop them at

any cost!

Dear Dementia,
I'm not a condition
I'm not an illness
I'm not a disease
I'm not a symptom

I'm Doris.

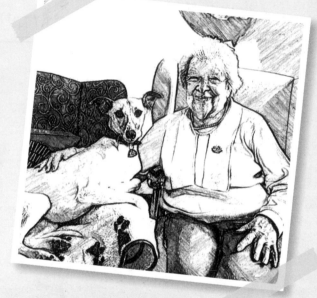

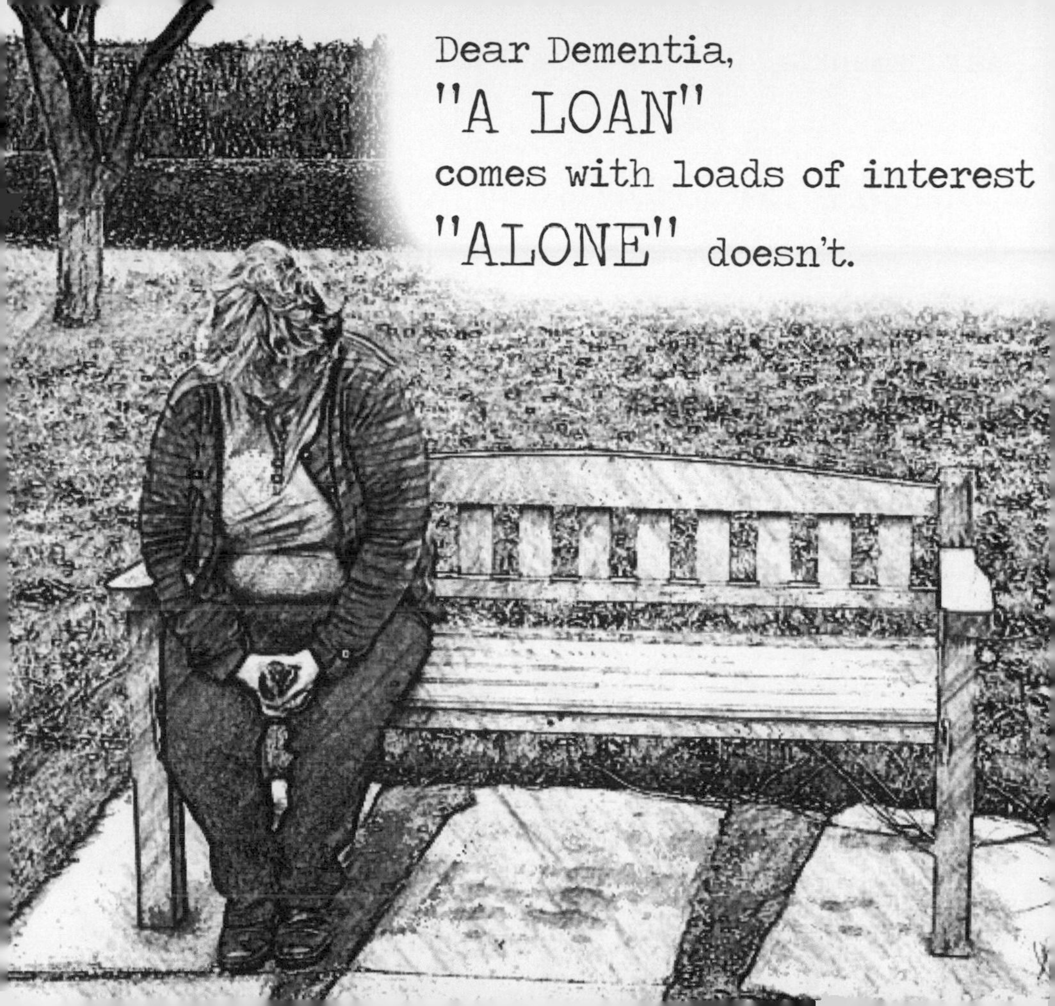

Dear Dementia,
"A LOAN"
comes with loads of interest
"ALONE" doesn't.

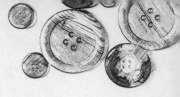

Dear Dementia,

I hate shopping nowadays.

"That'll be £15.67"

I hold my hand out and hope for the best.

Take my money, give me my shopping,
give me my change.

No questions please.

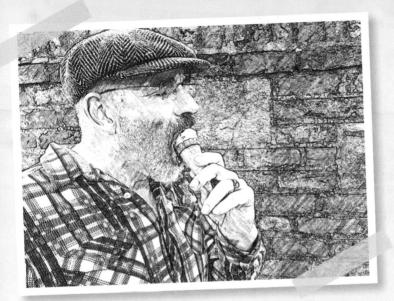

Dear Dementia,

Please stop Dad getting
on a train to Blackpool.

He lives in Bradford.

Not again...

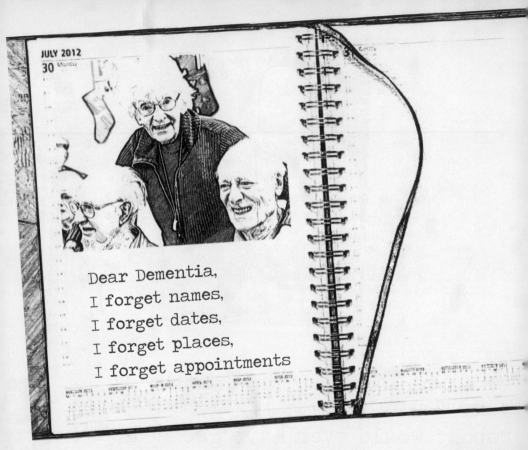

JULY 2012
30 Monday

Dear Dementia,
I forget names,
I forget dates,
I forget places,
I forget appointments

...Please don't forget ME!

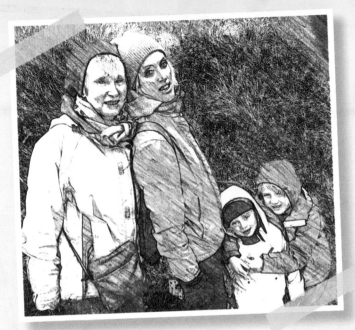

Dear Dementia,

Had a lovely family day at the seaside.
Fish and chips, ice cream, paddling in the sea.

Nobody would ever have guessed
you were with us!

Dear Dementia,

Time = numbers

Date = numbers

Telephones = numbers

Money = numbers

Cooking = numbers

I don't have numbers

I have YOU

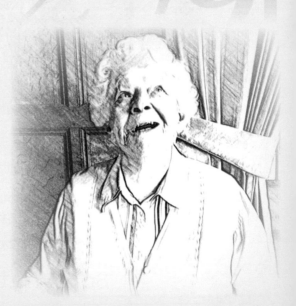

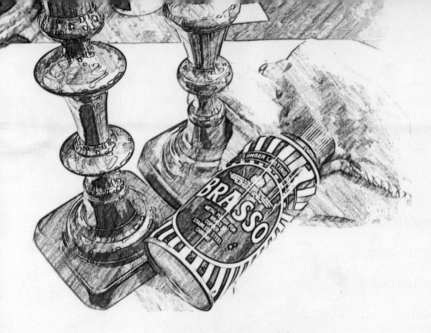

Dear Dementia,

She picks out my clothes,
washes me, dresses me, makes my bed,
cleans my room and ties my laces

So... What do I do, again?

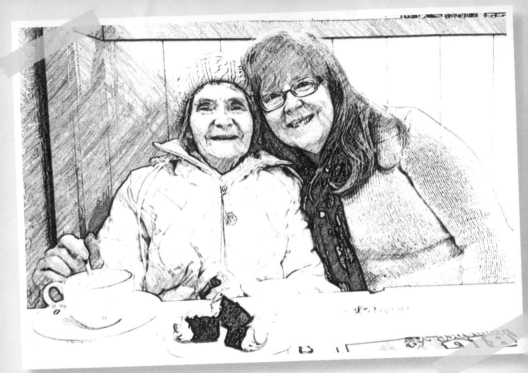

Dear Dementia,

I sacrificed everything to give my daughter the career she deserved. Now she's sacrificed her career for me. It was never meant to be a LOAN.

Dear Dementia,

I love that what's-his-name Barker off
The Two Ronnies

Dear Dementia,

Went to the Doctor today. She said I had problems with my cognitive skills and had issues with my parietal lobe and occipital lobe. I can't have you or else she'd never use such confusing words. Would she?

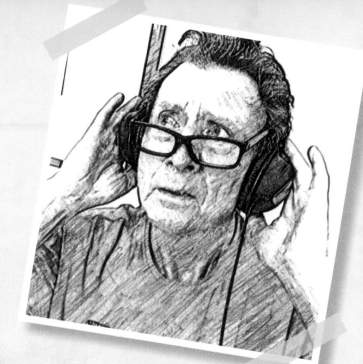

Dear Dementia,

I've just heard

"Keep young and beautiful
if you want to be loved"

on the radio. I used to love that song.

Not so keen today.

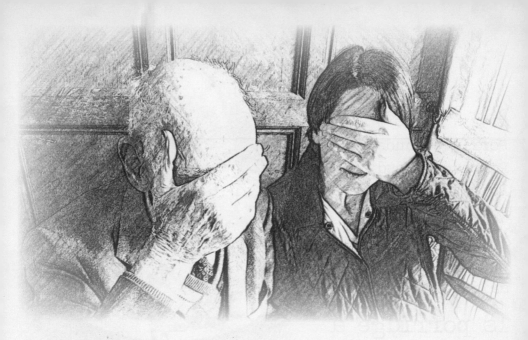

Dear Dementia,

I bathed Dad with my eyes closed today.
For him.
For me.
For dignity.
Please tell me when we can open our eyes?

Dear Dementia,

Porridge Monday
Porridge Tuesday
Porridge Wednesday
Porridge every
bloody day

I wish I'd never
said I like porridge.

Is porridge a
cure for you?

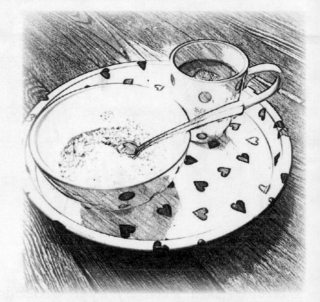

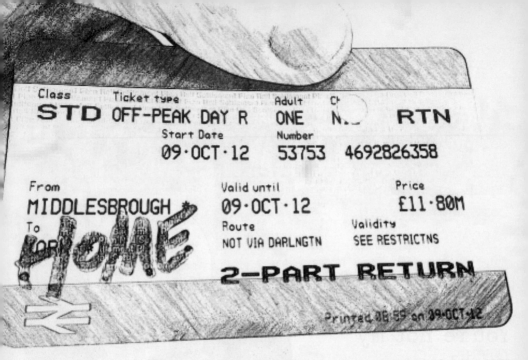

Dear Dementia,

"Can I have a single ticket please?"
"Where would you like to go sir?"

"Home"

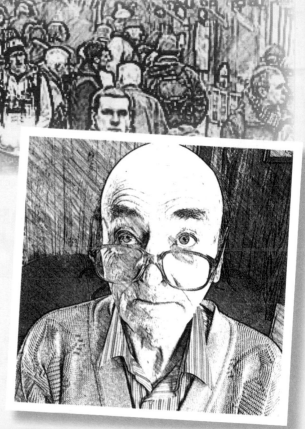

Dear Dementia,

You're not my problem.

Other people are!

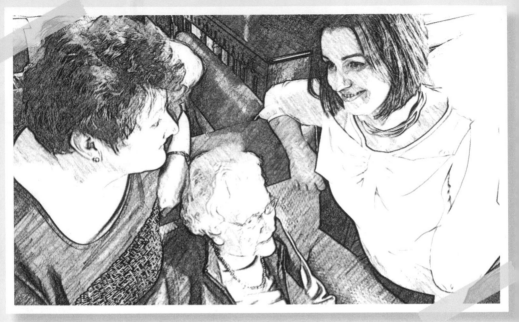

Dear Dementia,

"Does SHE take sugar?"
"Does SHE like porridge?"
"Does SHE want to go out?"
Have you made me INVISIBLE?

Have I disappeared?

Dear Dementia,
In France I'm "une homme vieux"
"A man who is old"
In English I'm an "old man"
Please see the MAN before the OLD
Merci!

Dear Dementia,
Keys?! Keys?! Keys?!
Bloody keys?!
You win that one
every time!

Dear Dementia,

I'm only called a **"wanderer"** because there's nothing to do.

If there was, I'd be called a **"gardener"** or **"painter"**

Dear Dementia,
I used to love to cook.
But cooking is numbers.
How many grams?
How many minutes?
How many degrees?

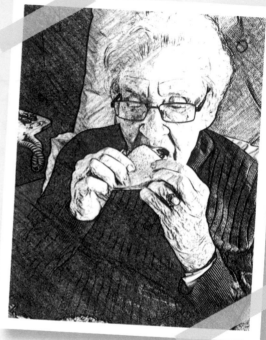

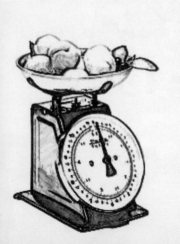

.....I think I'll make
a sandwich.

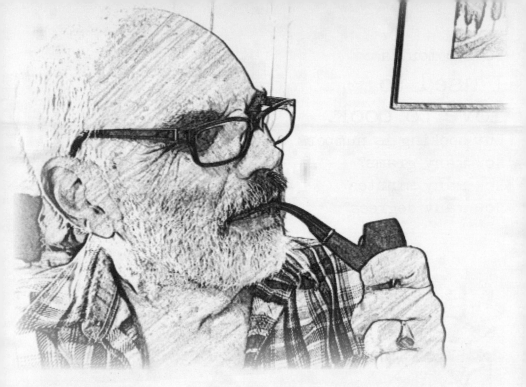

Dear Dementia,
I'm so glad that they always remember;
they work in my home
I don't live in their workplace.

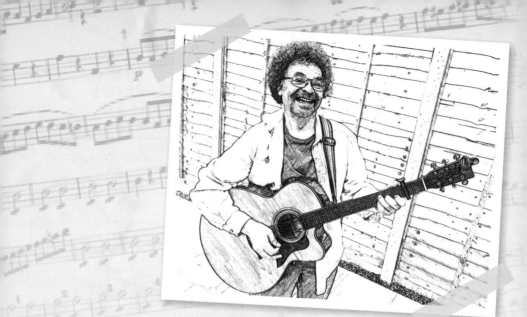

Dear Dementia,
When I look for words
many have gone.
When I try to find names
they've gone too.
But music remains.

Thanks for leaving me music.

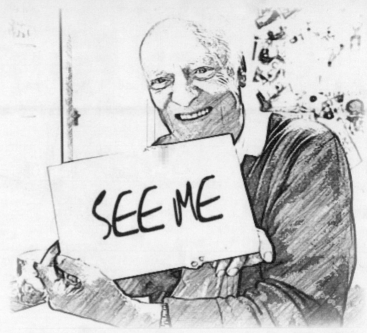

Dear Dementia,
I used to tremble with fear when my homework
had those two terrifying words

"See Me".

I wish more people would "SEE ME".

Instead they **"Could do better".**

Dear Dementia,
My blister pack
starts on Thursday.

When's
Thursday?

Dear Dementia,

"Keith, can you count
down from 100 to 0?"

"Can you spell
HOUSE backwards?"

"What shape is
the odd one out?"

Can't they do it?
Doctors used to be
cleverer in my day.

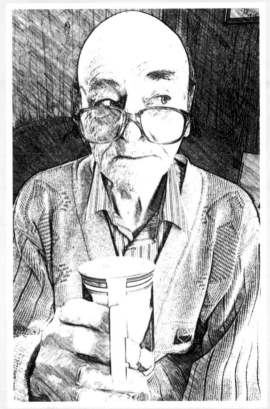

Dear Dementia,

I'm stuck on my desert island

A boat arrives

They help me for 10 minutes

Write about me for 5 minutes

Then jump back on the boat

Please come back soon...

Dear Dementia,

When Nana looks after me

She is happy

At the same time I sort
of look after Nana
and that makes me happy.

We love our
girls' nights in

Nana

Anni

Lu lu!

I Rnow I'm amazing

Dear Dementia,
Visitors don't use our cups.
Care staff don't use our cups.
What's wrong with us again?

Are you contagious?

Dear Dementia,
If they put a blank
piece of paper
on my door

what could they
write about me?

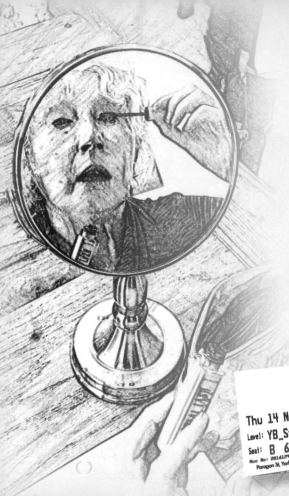

Dear Dementia,

I'm off to see Bryan Ferry tonight.

I'm leaving you at home in case you cramp my style.

I'm taking a change of underwear and my toothbrush just in case.

Don't wait up!

SJM Concerts and Live Nation Present

An Evening With

BRYAN FERRY

Thu 14 Nov 2013   Doors: 6:30 pm

Level: YB_Stalls Side Right Door: Right Area: Side

Seat: B 6   Price: £65.00 Adv

Acc No: 2016127 STennant 03/12/12 (*) Full   Order No: 180234392

Paragon St, York YO10 4NT   Box Office: 0844 854 2757   www.yorkbarbicon.co.uk

BARBIC

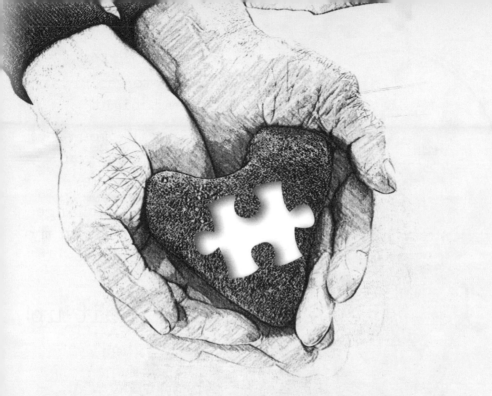

Dear Dementia,
Not even charity shops want jigsaw
puzzles with missing pieces.

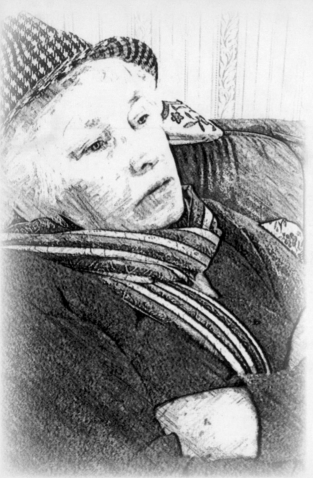

Dear Dementia,

My new care home copied my old front door.

I thought it was a lovely idea.

But every time I open it, it promises so much and delivers only heartbreak.

Dear Dementia,
Heart attack? Survived.
Cancer? Beat it.
Dementia? Work in progress.

Dear Dementia,
Total strangers undress me,
shower me and put me to bed
without introducing themselves.
Lasses never used to be so forward.

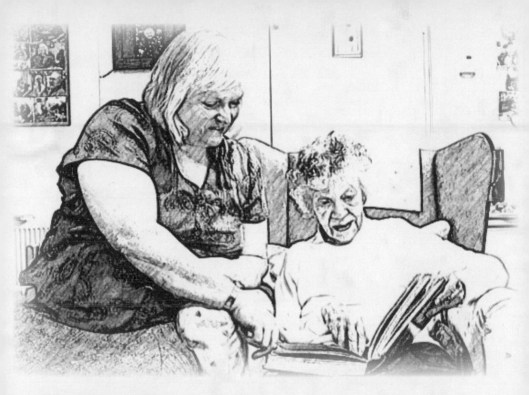

Dear Dementia,
Thanks for not stealing my ability to read yet.
But I've been reading lots of books about you and
NONE have a happy ending.

Dear Dementia,

I used to feel sorry
for animals in zoos.

People would come and
talk about them through
a pane of glass.

No animal deserves that.

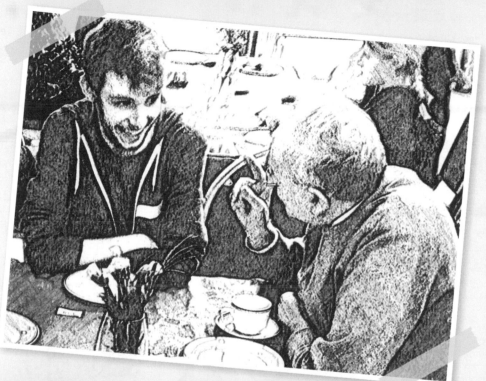

Dear Dementia,
Apathy? Never.
Sympathy? No thanks.
Empathy? That's the one!

Dear Dementia,
Going for a meal with the family. I can't wait to see them. I hope we talk about ME and THEM all day.

NOT about you!

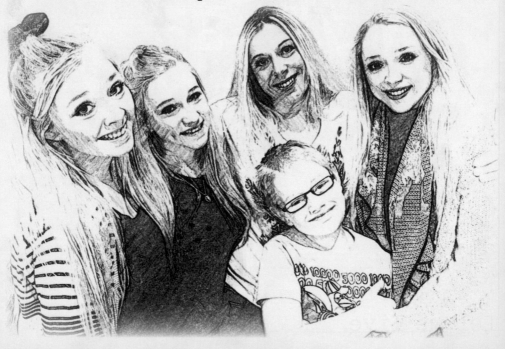

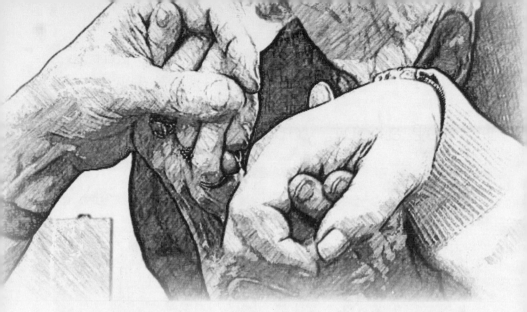

Dear Dementia,
It's hard to breathe when wrapped
in cotton wool.
Let me try.
Let me fail.
Let me succeed.

Let me live.

Dear Dementia,
I've been alive for
74 years,
raised 4 children,
had 11 grandchildren,
yet
no one knows
what size
shoes I wear.

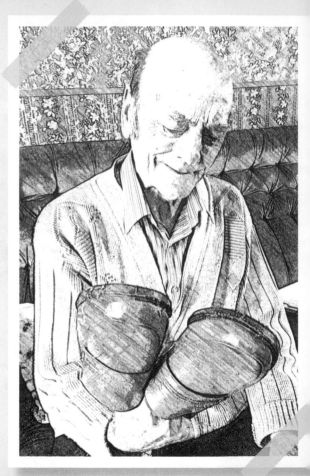

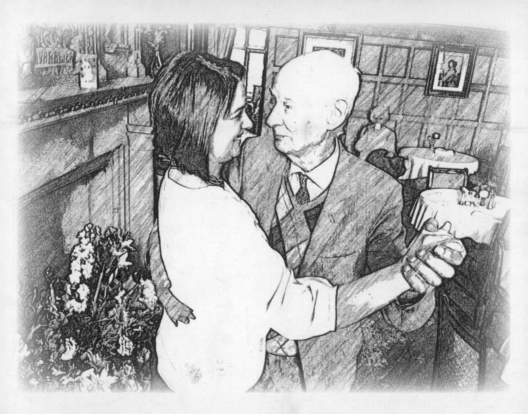

Dear Dementia,
The same heart beat inside of me when I
was 5, 25, 45 and 95. The same heart. The same ME.

Dear Dementia,
Dad was our hero.
He'd protect us from everything.
He'd climb the tallest trees to rescue us.
I wish he could save us from you.
But you've conquered our hero.

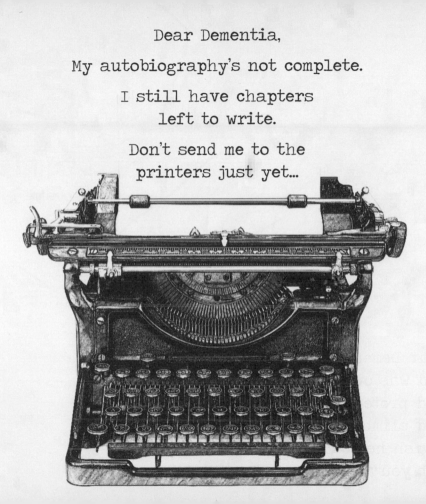

Dear Dementia,

My autobiography's not complete.

I still have chapters
left to write.

Don't send me to the
printers just yet...

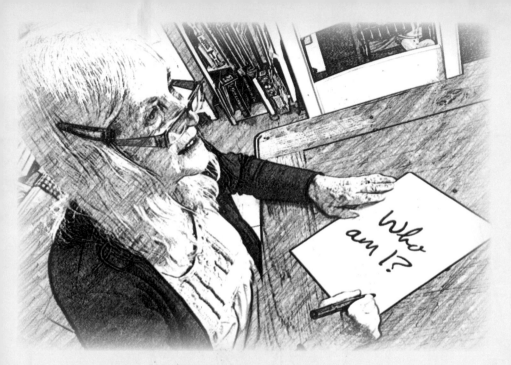

Dear Dementia,
In hospital I'm a patient.
In a care home I'm a service-user.
In respite I'm a guest.

Who am I again?

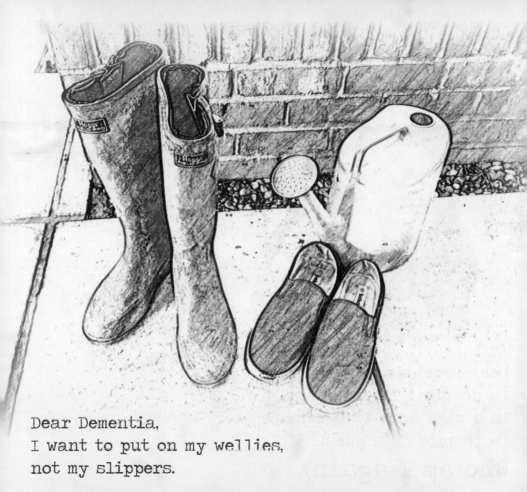

Dear Dementia,
I want to put on my wellies,
not my slippers.

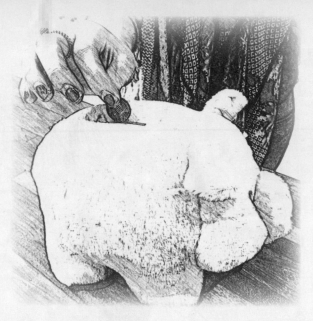

Dear Dementia,
The hole in the wall has eaten my cash card.
They won't give me it back.
Pin numbers?
Passwords?
Secret questions?
I wish I'd kept my piggy bank.

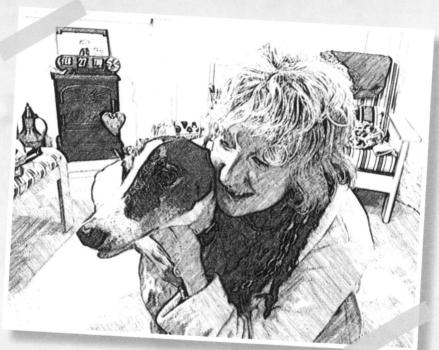

Dear Dementia,
Having Lulu is wonderful. She's companion, friend, exercise, fresh air, she reminds me to eat and people always talk to us. Without her I'd probably not bother, and you'd win.

Dear Dementia,
How can people
respect my
wishes if they
don't know them?
Ask.

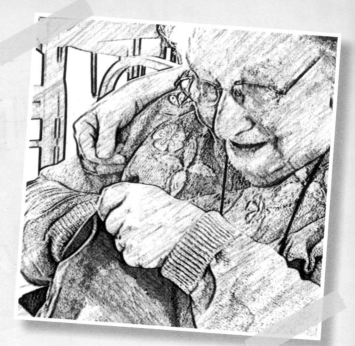

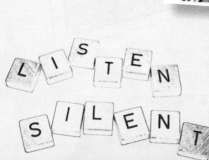

Dear Dementia,
If your favourite shop hasn't
had a delivery for some time,
lots of the 'good stuff' would have gone.
And only odd items remain.
Still shop there. They need your custom.

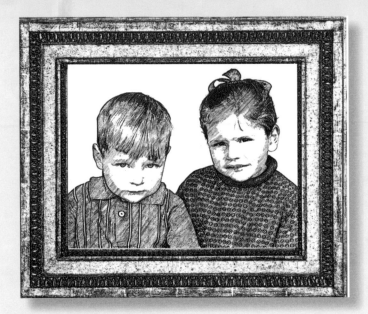

Dear Dementia,
If we replaced
"people with Dementia"
with the word "Children"
and the poor way they are
treated, there would be uproar.

Dear Dementia,

I can still read words fine.

The mechanics of reading are still there.

But I don't absorb any of it.

I'll save a fortune on books

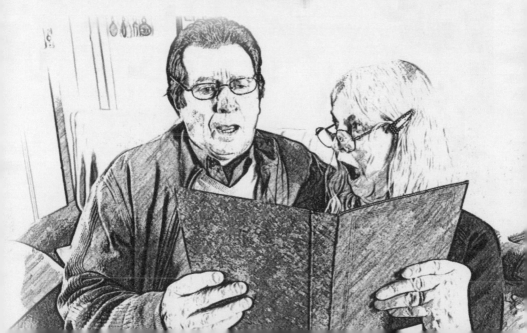

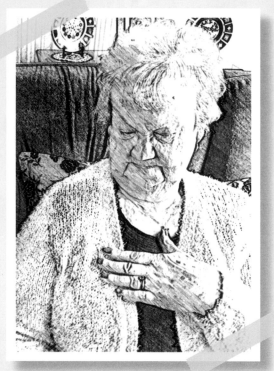

Dear Dementia,
Norah called me a
thief today.
My house - my cardigan.
My house - my mug.
My house - my teeth.
They suit me better
anyway.

Dear Dementia,
I hit Audrey today.
I've never hit her before.
I'd never hit her.
Did I hit her?
Did you hit her?
Or did we?

Dear Dementia,

I saw that nice man again today.

I don't know his name, but I know that I love him.

Dear Dementia,

Having you with me is like playing

'snakes and ladders'

But you've stolen all the ladders.

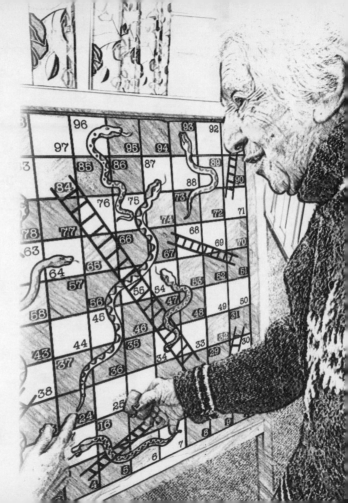

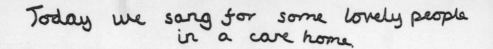

Today we sang for some lovely people in a care home.

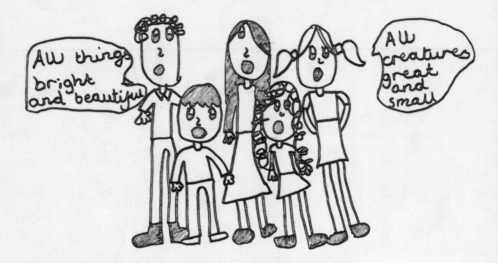

Dear Dementia,
A **primary school choir** came to sing today. We loved it. They couldn't see you.

They just saw us.

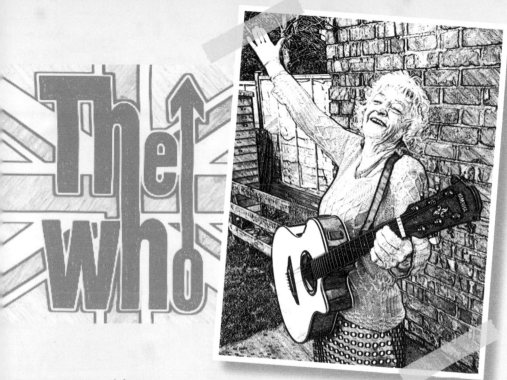

The Who

Dear Dementia,
I'm tired of Vera Lynn telling me 'We'll meet again' and about the colour of Dover's cliffs. Do you have anything by The Who?

Dear Dementia,
Thanks for
showing me
who my true
friends are.

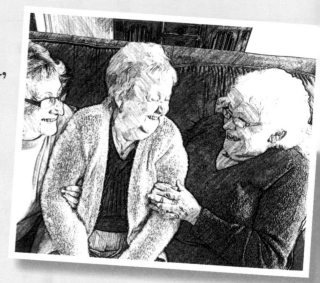

Dear Dementia,
We have a big family.
You've only got Dad so far.
Why do I only see my footprints in the sand
whilst the rest bury their heads in it
hoping you'll just go away?

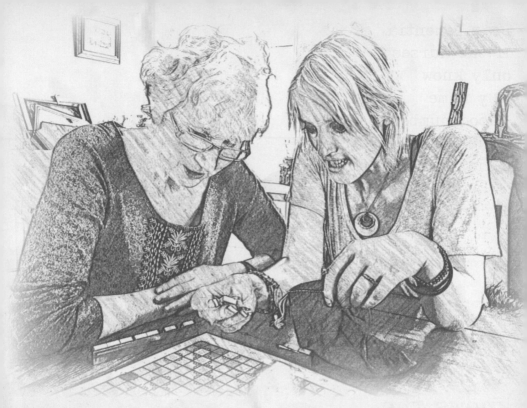

Dear Dementia,
There is no 'U' in 'lonely'
There's only ME.

Dear Dementia,
If the nurses
only knew
- My name
- Room number
- What I eat and drink
- What I look like.

A farmer
knows the
same about
his cows!

Dear Dementia,
There's always
a reason
why I do things
**please look
for it.**

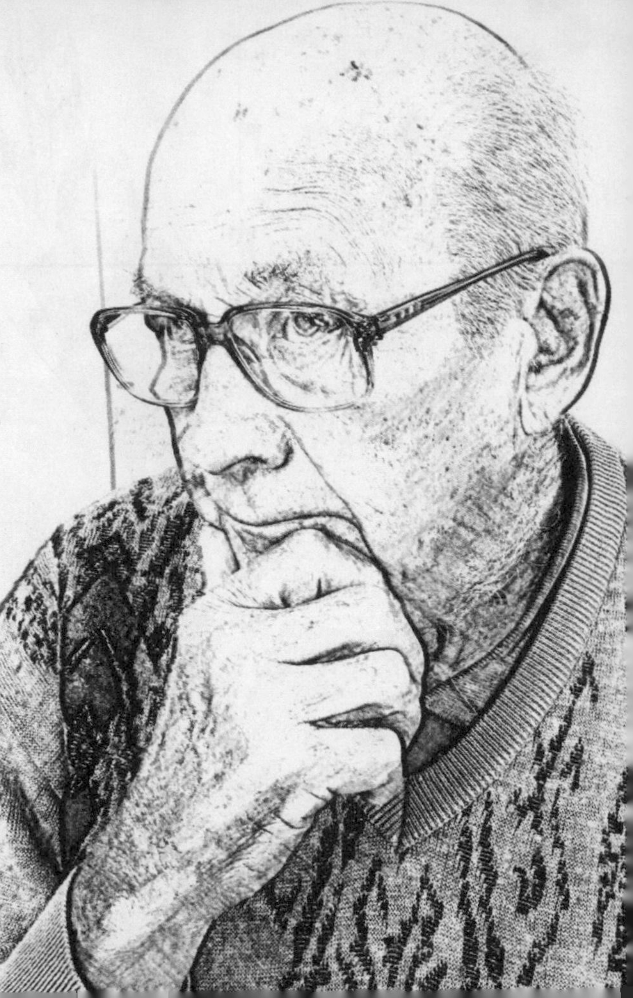

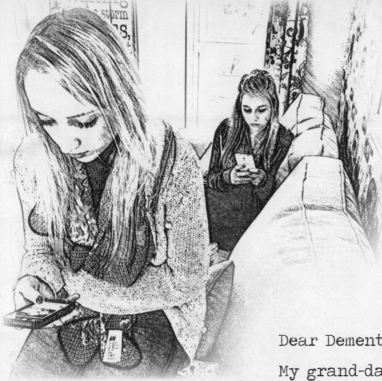

Dear Dementia,

My grand-daughter must be a genius at Maths.

She's always tapping away on her calculator these days.

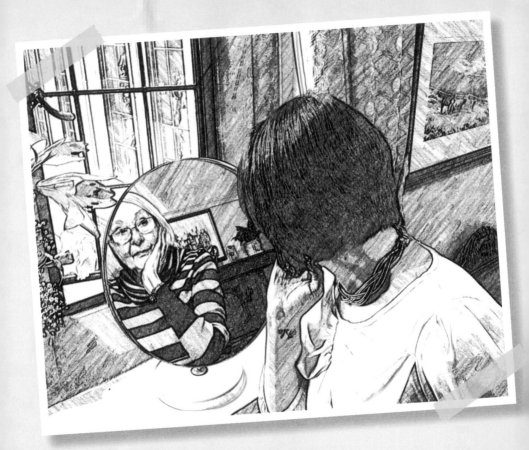

Dear Dementia,

I'm 25, yet people talk to
me like I'm an old woman.

I saw that lady
again today.

I wonder who she is?

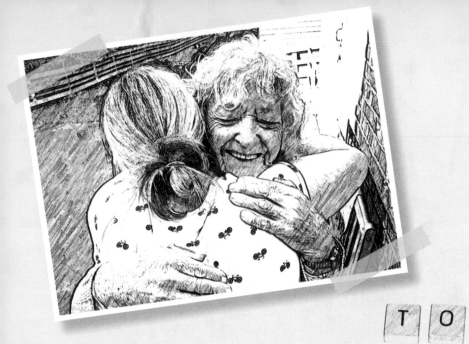

Dear Dementia,
If you've come for our mother
you may struggle
TO-GET-HER
because we are TOGETHER!

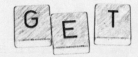

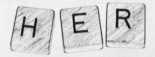

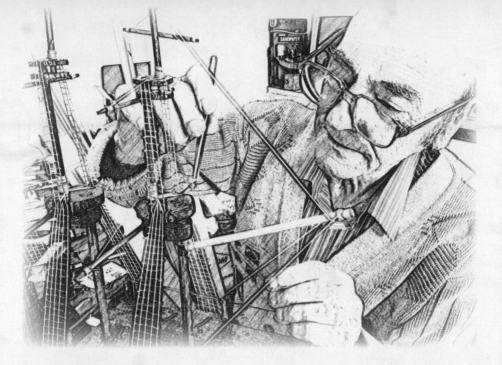

Dear Dementia,

I was born in a time when if something was broken you fixed it, you didn't throw it away.

I wish I could fix you.

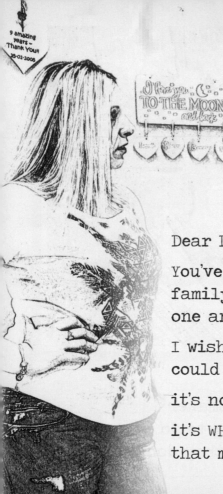
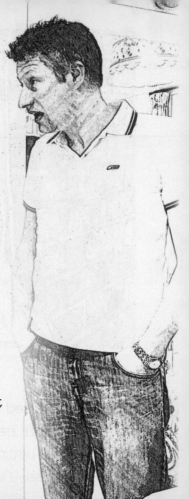

Dear Dementia,

You've turned my family against one another.

I wish they could see

it's not WHO'S right

it's WHAT's right that matters.

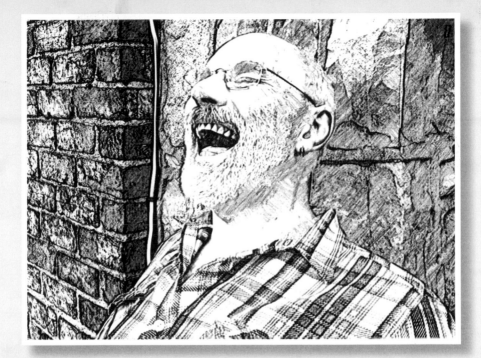

Dear Dementia,
Ida in Room 6 used to be a dressmaker
so they've given her some sewing to do.
I used to be a bouncer - I hope they don't expect me to
break up fights. I'm 76!

Dear Dementia,
You will win the war
eventually.
But we have many
battles to win between
now and then!

Thank you all for being truly invaluable
I know I will forget some people so forgive me...

All at Alzheimer's Support Wiltshire.

The line drawings in much of this book are based on photographs by Grant Newton taken at Alzheimer's Support's day club in Devizes, Wiltshire.

www.trainingforcarers.co.uk

Cherie Bakewell
- my wonderful designer

Alison, Kevin and all at Peregrine House

Gill, Tony and all at Riccall Carers

Jane, Wendy and all Barnsley Dementia Champions

Lou Squires and all the Millings and St. John's House

Jill Shearer and all at MMCG

Di and all at the Hall

Mike Padgham and all at the ICG

Brian McGuire and team at Visioncall

Yorkshire Ambulance

All Dementia Champions

Tommy and Joan Whitelaw

Bluebird Care

Chris Roberts and Jayne Goodrick

Tony's infectious smile and
the music within him

Pam and Lucy and all at
Grimston Court

York Harmony Dementia Café

Hannah and Michael

Kim Pennock

Liz, Emma, Annie, Billy, Lulu

Graham Hodge

Andrew and Di and Team
Wadell-Brown

Charlie Donaghy

Anna Oulton

Alison and Claire at
the Coach House

Leonnie Martin

Claire Tester

Everybody who gave their
time for nothing at
'A Night to Remember'

Keith, Vince and Agnes
from Tow Law

Auntie Jennie, Beryl and Renee

For your artistic and creative
input - Keara Stewart, Andy G and
Steve Barnsley

Trevor Jarvis BEM EDE

Simone & all at Woodlands

Kjartan Poskitt

The warm hearted Suzy Webster
and Alive Tim who don't know how
amazing they are

But most of all to the amazing
people living with dementia who
enrich my life every day just by
talking to me

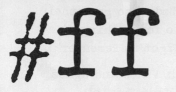

#ff

Twitter is a tremendous community for help and advice when caring for someone living with dementia.

Here are some amazing friends to follow who inspire and share their wonderful ideas with warmth and care. Thank you all.

Follow me
@TrainingCarers

@tommyNtour
@nurse_w_glasses
@suzysopenheart
@dragonmisery
@WhoseShoes
@mason4233
@SarahReed_MHR
@KimSea2shore
@Mike_Padgham
@McCayPaul
@nursemaiden
@wilfwardfamtst
@DAAcarers
@bethybl886

@legalaware
@N_Wilson94
@RoseHarwoodl
@KateSwaffer
@MrDarrenGormley
@CTrying
@MsLizStrange
@docofagesSophie
@edaming
@Chill4usCarers
@memorytriggers
@EngagingEmma
@PurpleAngelOrg
@verdigaldring
@IRememberBetter
@JeremyHughesAlz
@soo_cchsc

@AlzSocYorkshire
@TPurpleElephant
@avanteceo
@SHensonAmphlett
@LadderMoon
@acorns47
@ChrisMoonW
@CaregivingCafe
@Kimbohud
@WandererKirsty
@eileenshepherd
@janehughescook
@RobStewart
@jan_mcl3
@Bridgeanne
@EileenHMurphy
@SocialCareHour

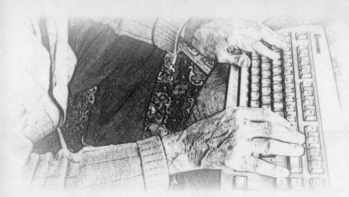

@jolivesleyl
@jeanniejuno
@trishteachermum
@TraceyJRobbins
@annatattonl
@KarenLisa66
@Andie_E
@NorthwayRuth
@keara_stewart
@joneslily65
@elinlowri
@meninsheds
@janeAnkori
@lpaice

@debsandsarah
@elucidate
@SamSherrington
@bronwynHemsley
@BrianSMcGuire
@NurChat
@dementia_2014
@TheRetreatYork
@jocrosslandbdg
@ProfBrendan
@EntwistleV
@dementia4school
@anniecoops
@ndowningl977

@val_hudson
@RominaOliverio
@SheelaghMachin
@dementiaadventure
@alzheimerssoc
@kenclemens
@weejoooon
@johnnyrockdogs
@Lorraine4Prep
@AnitaRolfe
@sallymagl
@JayneCooper100
@kenhowarduk
@christheeaglel
@DiverseAlz
@TommyTommyteel8
@xtraspirit
@Grow_Potential
@visioncall
@alivetim
@aliveactivities
@edanaming
@KarimS3D